STEADY HANDS STEADY MIND

Mindfulness for Surgeons in High-Stress Specialties

Dr MK Reddy

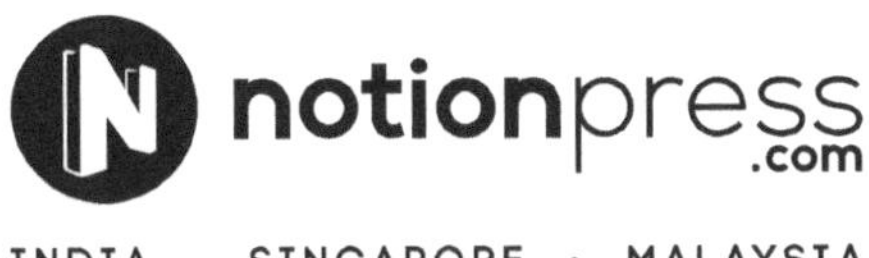

INDIA • SINGAPORE • MALAYSIA

ISBN 979-8-89929-397-9

For My Parents

Who are backbone to me in every aspect of my life

Contents

Foreword

If you've ever felt the intense pressure of making life-changing decisions, staying calm during emergencies, or simply trying to keep up with the demands of medical life, *"Steady Hands, Steady Mind"* is a book you need. It's a supportive and practical guide for healthcare professionals who want to stay mentally strong, emotionally balanced, and focused—even when the pressure is high and the days are long.

In a world where healthcare demands are rising and the pace of practice feels relentless, the emotional and cognitive toll on doctors, nurses, and frontline professionals has never been higher. Precision is non-negotiable. The stakes are human lives. And yet, amid the skill, speed, and service, one critical element is often overlooked: **the mental and emotional health of the healer.**

As a Mind Performance Coach and author of *"Unleash the Power of Reading,"* I've worked with countless professionals under extreme cognitive load—entrepreneurs, high-performing executives, and yes, doctors. Across all fields, the message is clear: **Burnout is real. But so is the way back.**

"Steady Hands, Steady Mind" beautifully blends mindfulness science with the lived reality of medical life. This book doesn't preach. It understands. It honors the grit of medical professionals while gently introducing practical, non-intrusive tools to regain clarity, focus, and emotional strength. From breathwork between procedures to mindfulness in the midst of trauma care, it shows how small shifts can create massive change—without requiring a sabbatical or retreat.

What makes this book truly special is its **balance of clinical understanding and human empathy.** Each chapter is filled with insight that is not only research-based but deeply relatable. It acknowledges the hidden pain behind depersonalization, the unspoken anxiety of young doctors in training, and the silent burnout that builds behind a brave face.

Whether you're a surgeon, an internist, an emergency physician, or a resident just beginning your journey, *"Steady Hands, Steady Mind"* offers a roadmap to help you stay sharp, present, and well—inside and outside the hospital walls.

This is more than a book on mindfulness. It is a lifeline for those who give everything, reminding them that their own mind and heart deserve care too.

To every healer reading this: **Your steadiness is your strength. Let this book help you protect it.**

Best wishes,

Manjunath MS

Mind Performance Coach | Author of *Unleash the Power of Reading*

Preface

In the world of surgery, precision is revered, focus is essential, and endurance is a quiet expectation. But beneath the steady hands that guide the scalpel lies an often-neglected truth—surgeons are human too. They bear not only the physical weight of long hours and high-stakes procedures but also the emotional strain of loss, responsibility, and relentless pressure.

"Steady Hands, Steady Mind" is a groundbreaking guide written not just from knowledge but from lived experience. This book is a compassionate companion for every surgical resident, practitioner, or healthcare professional who has felt the emotional turbulence that often lies hidden behind the calm façade of the OR.

With clarity, empathy, and remarkable insight, the author bridges the gap between surgical science and mental well-being. From practical mindfulness tools and stress management techniques to emotional resilience and work-life balance, every chapter serves as both mirror and medicine—helping readers reflect, recover, and realign.

This is more than a self-help manual. It is a manifesto for a new kind of surgeon—one who leads with both skill and self-awareness. A surgeon who listens to patients and to themselves. A professional who doesn't just survive the storm but learns to dance in the rain.

If you're ready to become that surgeon, this book is your first step. Read it with an open heart, and it will not only sharpen your scalpel but also strengthen your spirit.

"A rare gem in medical literature."

"Blends science, psychology, and lived experience into something profoundly human. The subtle humor makes the heavy topics feel lighter and relatable."

Dr K Manohar Melchizedek

MS (General Surgery)

Assistant Professor, Guntur Medical College

"A must-read for every surgeon with a beating heart."

"This book brings balance to a world where we often forget ourselves while saving others. It's a reminder that mental clarity is as vital as clinical skill."

Dr Chandra Mohan Prakash

MS (General Surgery)

Assistant Professor, Guntur Medical College

"The book I wish I had in my first year of residency."

"The mindfulness techniques are so doable—even between cases. The writing feels like a mentor gently guiding you through the chaos of surgical life."

Dr Uday Bhaskar Chandu

MS (General Surgery)

"Helped me reconnect with why I became a doctor."

"The sections on mindful communication and maintaining personal identity are brilliant. It's healing, practical, and surprisingly inspiring."

Prof Sreekanth Kumar Mallineni

BDS, PGDip, MDS, Adv Dip DSPaediatrDent, (PhD)

1.   **Introduction: The Journey of a Surgeon**

Purpose and scope of the book.

The unique demands and rewards of a career in surgery.

The importance of mental clarity, resilience, and self-care for long-term success.

2.   **Chapter 1: The Realities of General Surgery Residency**

◆   Common challenges faced by surgical residents (e.g., long hours, high stakes, emotional toll).

◆   Statistics and case studies on burnout, stress, and mental health issues among surgeons.

◆   Setting realistic expectations for life as a surgical resident.

3.   **Chapter 2: An Introduction to Mindfulness**

◆   Defining mindfulness and its core principles.

◆   Scientific evidence and research supporting mindfulness in high-stress professions.

◆   Key benefits for surgeons: improved focus, patience, empathy, and stress reduction.

4.   **Chapter 3: Practical Mindfulness Techniques for Surgeons**

◆   Techniques that fit into the demanding schedule of a surgeon (e.g., breathing exercises, guided meditation).

◆   Applying mindfulness in preoperative and postoperative settings.

◆   Real-time strategies for staying present during high-stress moments.

5.   **Chapter 4: Managing Stress in the OR and Beyond**

◆   Recognizing the signs and symptoms of acute and chronic stress.

◆ Techniques to cope with stress in high-stakes environments, like surgeries and emergencies.

◆ Long-term resilience-building habits, from reflective journaling to mindfulness-based stress reduction.

6. **Chapter 5: Building Emotional Resilience**

◆ Understanding emotional resilience and its importance in surgery.

◆ Tools for managing emotions during challenging cases.

◆ Methods to develop compassion and empathy without experiencing burnout.

7. **Chapter 6: Maintaining Physical and Mental Health**

◆ Importance of physical fitness and its effect on mental clarity and stamina.

◆ Strategies for regular exercise, sleep hygiene, and balanced nutrition in a busy schedule.

◆ Techniques for maintaining mental health, including therapy, peer support, and self-care routines.

8. **Chapter 7: Balancing Professional and Personal Life**

◆ Defining work-life balance and setting boundaries.

◆ Practical tips for scheduling personal time, family time, and rest.

◆ Using mindfulness to reduce guilt and stay present during personal time.

9. **Chapter 8: Patient Interaction with Mindfulness and Empathy**

◆ Techniques to communicate compassionately with patients and their families.

◆ Strategies for handling difficult patient interactions and emotionally intense cases.

◆ Incorporating empathy and mindfulness into bedside manner and patient counseling.

10. **Chapter 9: Building a Support System in Residency**

◆ The role of mentors, colleagues, family, and friends.

◆ How to create and nurture a network that supports mental well-being.

◆ Tips for leaning on peers during shared challenges and learning to ask for help.

11. **Chapter 10: Cultivating Hobbies and Interests Outside Medicine**

◆ How personal interests and hobbies can improve mental well-being.

◆ Encouraging surgical residents to pursue creative outlets and maintain a life outside the hospital.

◆ Balancing surgical identity with personal identity.

12. **Chapter 11: Preparing for Post-Residency Life**

◆ Planning a career that balances professional goals and personal well-being.

◆ Transitioning from residency to practice with healthy coping mechanisms.

◆ Continuing mindfulness and stress management practices throughout a surgical career.

13. **Conclusion: Steady Hands, Steady Mind**

◆ Recap of the key takeaways from each chapter.

◆ Final encouragement for readers to prioritise mental and physical well-being.

◆ The ongoing journey of mindfulness in a life-long surgical career.

Introduction

Surgical residency is not only a journey of mastering skills but also one of developing unbreakable mental and emotional strength. In the high-stakes environment of the operating room (OR), every decision is critical, every movement matters, and every mistake is magnified. Surgeons are expected to be pillars of calm and precision. Yet, beneath the surface, the realities of residency—long hours, intense stress, physical fatigue, and emotional strain—challenge even the most resilient individuals. This book is written for you, the surgical resident or practising surgeon, navigating these unique demands with courage and dedication.

In *Steady Hands, Steady Mind*, we embark on mastering mindfulness in high-stress surgical specialities. Mindfulness has gained recognition as a tool for stress relief and a powerful method to enhance focus, clarity, and emotional resilience. Studies have shown that mindfulness reduces burnout, improves patient interactions, and sharpens cognitive skills—all essential qualities for any surgeon. However, the **application of mindfulness in the surgical field is still evolving**, and its potential for surgeons is vast. This book offers a structured approach to integrating mindfulness and self-care into your practice, helping you become a surgeon with not only steady hands but also a steady mind.

Why Mindfulness for Surgeons?

Mindfulness, the practice of being present and fully engaged in the moment, is especially valuable in surgery, where intense focus and a calm demeanour are essential. High-stress situations can cloud judgment and affect performance, but you can learn to maintain clarity under pressure by honing mindfulness techniques. This book will provide a variety of mindfulness practices tailored specifically for surgeons, from grounding exercises for the OR to stress-relief techniques post-surgery.

Overview of the Book

The following chapters will cover topics crucial for surgical professionals facing high demands, providing tools and insights to support your mental and emotional well-being:

1. **Understanding the Challenges of Surgical Residency**

   We'll start with an honest look at the pressures you face daily and how these impact mental health, work-life balance, and resilience.

2. **Practical Mindfulness Techniques**

   You'll learn simple yet powerful mindfulness exercises, including breathing techniques, visualisations, gratitude and grounding practices designed to be integrated seamlessly into your busy schedule.

3. **Mental Health and Emotional Resilience**

   This section explores recognising and addressing signs of burnout, managing performance anxiety, and building emotional strength to stay grounded through intense challenges.

4. **Work-Life Balance in the OR and Beyond**

   We'll explore strategies to help you balance your demanding professional life with personal time, relationships, and self-care, helping you create a sustainable, fulfilling life.

5. **Navigating Patient and Family Interactions Mindfully**

   Enhancing communication with patients and their families can create positive outcomes for both you and those in your care.

This chapter discusses empathy, compassionate communication, and boundary-setting to support both patient care and personal well-being.

6.   **Staying Resilient: Post-Residency Life and Beyond**

Transitioning from residency to practice presents new challenges. You'll find insights on maintaining well-being and mindfulness throughout your surgical career.

Steady Hands, Steady Mind offers a guide to transform your practice with intention, focus, and resilience. As we journey through each chapter, my hope is that you find support, insight, and tools that empower you to thrive in both your personal and professional life. Whether you're scrubbing in for a complex procedure, debriefing after a long day, or striving for balance at home, let this book be your companion on the journey to becoming not only a skilled surgeon but a mindful, resilient one.

1

The Realities of General Surgery Residency

Introduction: The Demands of Surgical Residency

The journey of a surgical resident is one of immense challenge and transformation. For many, it is a rite of passage into one of the most demanding and rewarding professions in medicine. Residents face long hours, the pressure of high-stakes decision-making, and the emotional toll of patient outcomes—all while striving to master surgical skills. This chapter explores the harsh realities of residency while offering guidance to navigate its challenges effectively.

Common Challenges Faced by Surgical Residents

✳   **Long Hours and Physical Fatigue:**

Surgical residents often work shifts exceeding 80 hours a week, with days starting before sunrise and ending well after sunset. Extended hours lead to physical exhaustion, reduced cognitive function, and a heightened risk of errors.

◆   *Example*: A resident might be on call for more than 24 hours, managing emergency cases and performing procedures with little to no rest.

*** Emotional Toll and Patient Care:**

The emotional challenges include breaking bad news to patients'
families, dealing with adverse outcomes, and coping with the
weight of patient mortality.

- *Real-life scenario*: A resident losing their first patient during
  surgery and grappling with feelings of guilt and inadequacy.

*** Learning Curve and Performance Pressure:**

Residents are expected to learn quickly and perform under
pressure, balancing patient care with their own self-doubt. The
need to stay updated with medical knowledge while practicing
clinical skills adds to the stress.

Burnout, Stress, and Mental Health Issues Among Surgical Residents

*** Defining Burnout:**

Burnout is characterised by emotional exhaustion,
depersonalisation, and a reduced sense of accomplishment.
It is prevalent among residents due to intense workloads and
insufficient recovery time.

- *Statistic*: According to a 2023 study in *JAMA Surgery*, 54%
  of surgical residents report experiencing burnout, and 20%
  consider leaving their training programs.

*** Mental Health Challenges:**

- **Stress and Anxiety**: Constantly facing life-or-death
  situations creates chronic stress, which can escalate into
  anxiety disorders.

- **Depression**: The lack of time for self-care and social
  connections often leads to feelings of isolation and sadness.

  - *Example*: A resident who internalizes mistakes, leading
    to negative self-talk and depressive symptoms.

Setting Realistic Expectations for Life as a Surgical Resident

✳   **Understanding the Commitment:**

Surgical residency is not a sprint but a marathon. Residents must accept that sacrifices are inevitable but can be managed with foresight and planning.

◆   *Perspective:* Acknowledge that struggles are part of growth and that perfection is not always achievable in training.

✳   **Balancing Professional and Personal Life:**

◆   **Time Management:** Allocate time for both professional responsibilities and personal life. This includes scheduling brief moments of rest, meals, and family connections.

⚔   *Tip:* Use a daily planner to set priorities and identify gaps where rest or self-care can be integrated.

✳   **Building Resilience Through Preparation:**

◆   Be proactive in learning about the challenges ahead. Speak with senior residents and mentors about their coping strategies.

⚔   *Question for Reflection:* "What specific habits can I develop today to prepare for the demands of tomorrow?"

Evidence-Based Strategies for Managing Residency Challenges

✳   **Mindfulness and Stress Management:**

Mindfulness practices can help residents stay present and reduce anxiety in high-pressure situations. Techniques include:

◆   *Deep Breathing:* A quick tool during stressful surgeries or patient interactions.wim-hoff

⚔   *Grounding Exercises:* Focus on the senses to calm the mind during moments of overwhelm.

5-4-3-2-1 technique for grounding exercise.

5 things you can see

4 things you can touch

3 things you can hear

2 things you can smell

1 emotion you can feel

Step-by-Step Explanation

1. **Five Things You Can See**

    ◆　Look around you and identify five things that you can visually observe.

    ◆　These could be objects in the room, people, shapes, colors, or even subtle details like light reflections or textures.

    ◆　Example: "I see a clock on the wall, my phone on the desk, the green plant by the window, the books on the shelf, and the pattern on the carpet."

    ◆　Why It Helps: Engaging your sense of sight forces your mind to focus outward, breaking the cycle of anxious thoughts.

2. **Four Things You Can Touch**

    ◆　Pay attention to four things you can physically feel around you.

    ◆　These can be objects you're holding, your clothes against your skin, the chair beneath you, or even the floor under your feet. If possible, physically touch them.

    ◆　Example: "I feel the smooth surface of my desk, the warmth of my coffee cup, the texture of my jeans, and the softness of the cushion I'm sitting on."

    ◆　Why It Helps: Engaging your sense of touch grounds you in the physical world, creating a sense of stability and safety.

3. **Three Things You Can Hear**

   ◆　Focus on three sounds in your environment.

   ◆　These could be external sounds (e.g., birds chirping, cars passing by, distant conversations) or internal sounds (e.g., your own breathing, the hum of a fan).

   ◆　Example: "I hear the ticking of the clock, the faint sound of traffic outside, and the rustling of papers on my desk."

   ◆　Why It Helps: Tuning into subtle auditory details shifts your focus from racing thoughts to your sensory surroundings.

4. **Two Things You Can Smell**

   ◆　Identify two scents in your environment.

   ◆　If you can't immediately notice any smells, try finding something with a scent (e.g., a nearby cup of tea, a scented candle, or even the smell of your own clothes).

   ◆　Example: "I smell the aroma of my coffee and the fresh scent of my hand lotion."

   ◆　Why It Helps: Smell has a powerful link to memory and emotion, and focusing on pleasant or neutral scents can help calm your mind.

5. **One Emotion You Can Feel**

   ◆　Name one emotion you are currently feeling.

   ◆　It could be something as simple as calm, frustration, relief, or joy. Acknowledge the emotion without judgment—just observe it.

   ◆　Example: "I feel a little anxious, but also a sense of relief that I'm taking control of this moment."

   ◆　Why It Helps: Recognizing your emotional state helps build emotional awareness and acceptance, which are key components of mindfulness.

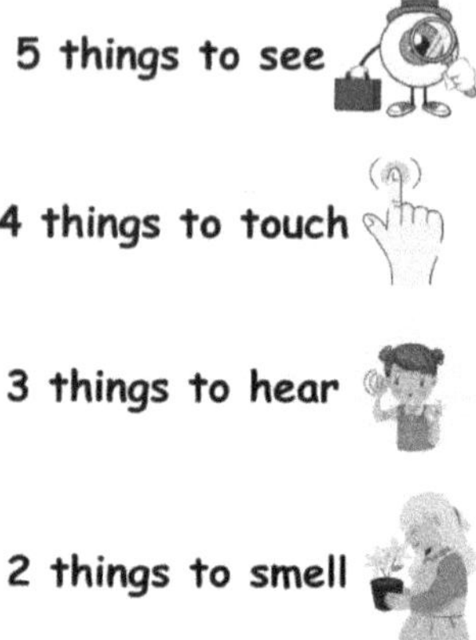

Why the 5-4-3-2-1 Technique Works

◆ Disrupts Negative Thought Patterns: By focusing on your senses, this technique interrupts cycles of anxiety or rumination.

◆ Promotes Mindfulness: It brings your awareness back to the present, rather than being stuck in the past or worrying about the future.

◆ Easy and Quick: It can be done anywhere, anytime, without the need for special tools or preparation.

Pro Tips for Practice

1. Practice Regularly: Even when you're not feeling stressed, practicing this technique can help you become more comfortable using it during high-stress situations.

2. Combine with Deep Breathing: Pairing the 5-4-3-2-1 exercise with slow, deep breaths enhances its calming effects.

3.　Adapt It to Your Needs: If certain senses are unavailable (e.g., you cannot smell anything at the moment), focus on other senses or repeat the exercise with additional items from a different sense.

✳　**Time Management and Efficiency**:

◆　**Prioritize Tasks**: Identify the most critical tasks to focus energy effectively.

◆　**Delegate and Collaborate**: Work closely with team members to share responsibilities.

⊿　*Example*: A resident reviewing patient charts the night before to save time during rounds.

✳　**Emotional Support Systems**:

◆　Build a network of mentors, peers, and mental health professionals.

⊿　*Action Point*: Schedule regular check-ins with a mentor or therapist to discuss challenges.

Reflecting on the Residency Journey

Emotional support system

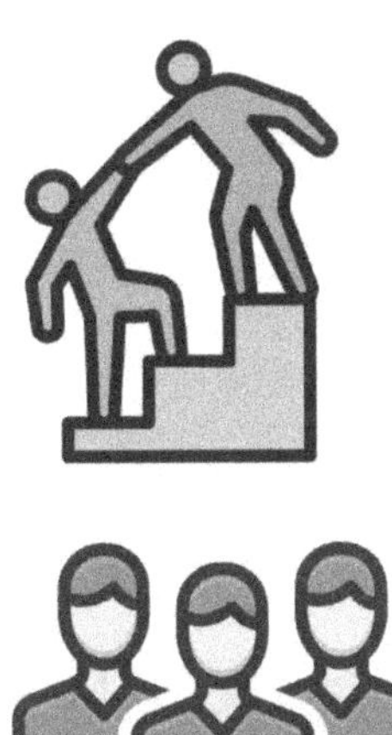

***   Recognising Growth Through Challenges**:

Each challenge presents an opportunity to grow both as a surgeon and as a person. Celebrate small wins, such as successfully assisting in a complex procedure or receiving gratitude from a patient's family.

***   Creating a Sustainable Career Path**:

- ◆   Focus on long-term goals while addressing immediate challenges.

- ◆   Learn to view setbacks as part of the learning curve rather than personal failures.

***   Looking Ahead**:

Prepare for post-residency life by envisioning the type of surgeon you want to become.

- ◆   *Prompt*: "What values will guide your practice as you transition from training to independent practice?"

Recap and Summary

Residency is not just about acquiring technical skills but about becoming a well-rounded surgeon who can handle the pressures of the profession. By recognizing the realities of residency and adopting evidence-based strategies, you can build a foundation for a fulfilling and sustainable career.

This detailed chapter offers a comprehensive understanding of the challenges faced by surgical residents while equipping them with actionable insights to navigate their journey effectively.

Key Points:

1.   Surgical residency is physically, mentally, and emotionally demanding, requiring resilience and adaptability.

2. Burnout and mental health challenges are prevalent but manageable through mindfulness, time management, and support systems.

3. Setting realistic expectations and prioritizing self-care can help residents thrive.

2

An Introduction to Mindfulness

Defining Mindfulness and Its Core Principles

What is Mindfulness?

Mindfulness is the practice of maintaining a moment-by-moment awareness of your thoughts, feelings, bodily sensations, and surrounding environment, free of judgment. It involves consciously paying attention to the present moment rather than dwelling on the past or worrying about the future.

Core Principles of Mindfulness:

1. **Awareness**: Observing your inner and outer world without bias.

2. **Acceptance**: Acknowledging experiences without labeling them as good or bad.

3. **Non-Judgment**: Letting go of critical thoughts and approaching situations with curiosity.

Actionable Insights:

✳   **Daily Practice**: Spend 5 minutes every morning focusing on your breath. Notice the air entering your nostrils and your chest rising and falling.

✳   **Mindfulness in Action**: Before starting a surgery, take 10 deep breaths to ground yourself and focus on the task ahead.

Mindfulness

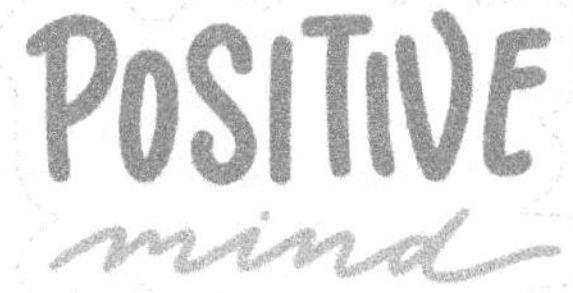

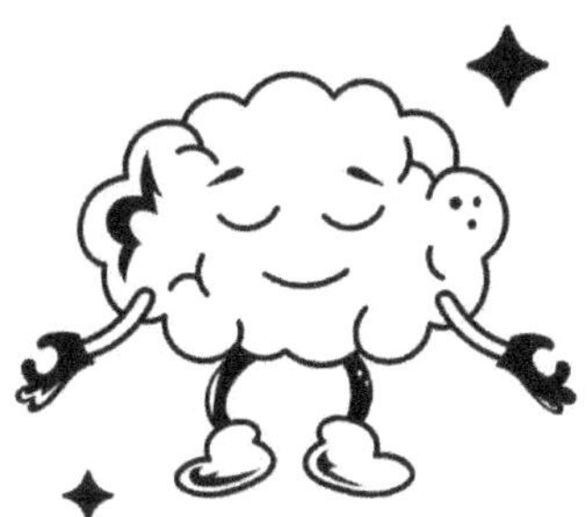

Interactive Element:

Reflection Prompt:

✳   "Think about the last time you felt overwhelmed. What thoughts were racing through your mind? How might observing these thoughts without judgment have changed your response?"

Scientific Evidence Supporting Mindfulness in High-Stress Professions

Research Findings:

* **Cognitive Benefits**: Studies show that mindfulness improves attention and working memory.

  * *Evidence*: A 2018 study in *Frontiers in Human Neuroscience* demonstrated that 8 weeks of mindfulness training led to significant improvements in sustained attention among healthcare professionals.

* **Emotional Regulation**: Mindfulness practices reduce the reactivity of the amygdala, the brain's emotional center, helping individuals respond more calmly to stress.

  * *Evidence*: Research published in *JAMA Internal Medicine* found that mindfulness meditation programs significantly reduced anxiety and depression in healthcare workers.

* **Physical Health**: Regular mindfulness practice lowers cortisol levels, reducing the physiological effects of stress.

Actionable Insights:

* A simplified program focusing solely on breathing techniques to manage stress and increase focus.

* **Core Elements**:

  * **4-7-8 Breathing**: Inhale for 4 counts, hold for 7 counts, exhale for 8 counts.

  * **Box Breathing**: Inhale, hold, exhale, and pause—each for 4 counts.

  * **Rescue Breaths**: Two slow, deep breaths to reset during moments of stress.

The STOP Technique

✳ **Description:**

A quick mindfulness exercise for pausing and refocusing during high-stress situations.

✳ **Core Elements:**

◆ **S:** Stop.

◆ **T:** Take a deep breath.

◆ **O:** Observe—acknowledge your thoughts, feelings, and body sensations.

◆ **P:** Proceed—resume with greater clarity and focus.

✳ **Relevance to Surgery:**

◆ Can be used between cases, during pre-op briefings, or after difficult situations.

Brain Accelerator Program by Dr Manjunath:

Its a beautiful and excellent program teaches mindfullness strategies to cope up day to day stress. You can enroll this program. It includes regular mindfulness sessions, explains how to be mindfull, selfhypnosis program, time management strategies, regulating emotions etc.

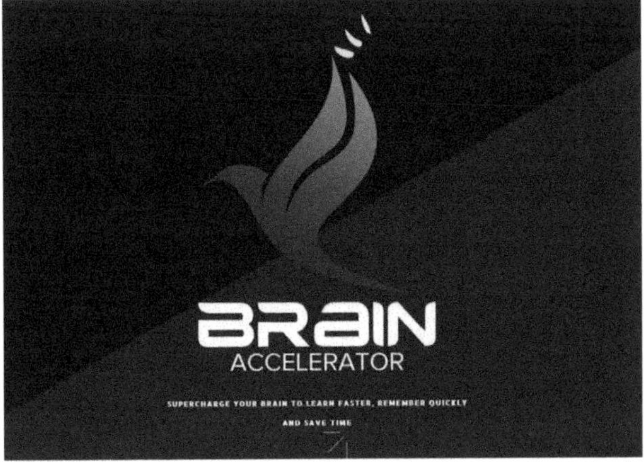

♦ Use mobile apps like *Headspace* or *Calm* for guided mindfulness sessions tailored for busy schedules.

Interactive Element:

Question:

* "What would it mean for you to have a clearer, calmer mind in the middle of a high-stakes surgery? How might this impact your decision-making and patient care?"

Benefits of Mindfulness for Surgeons

1. **Improved Focus and Attention:**

   ♦ Surgeons must maintain laser-like focus during procedures. Mindfulness trains the brain to sustain attention and avoid distractions.

      ⚔ *Example*: A surgeon who practices mindfulness before a procedure is better equipped to handle unexpected complications calmly.

2. **Enhanced Patience and Emotional Resilience:**

   ♦ In high-pressure environments, patience is essential. Mindfulness reduces impulsive reactions and fosters thoughtful responses.

      ⚔ *Scenario*: During a prolonged surgery, mindfulness can help you remain patient with both the process and the team.

3. **Increased Empathy and Better Patient Interactions:**

   ♦ Mindfulness helps surgeons connect with their patients on a deeper level, improving communication and trust.

      ⚔ *Example*: A surgeon practicing mindful listening can empathize with a patient's fears and provide reassurance more effectively.

4. **Stress Reduction:**

   ❖ Mindfulness decreases cortisol levels, helping surgeons manage the stress of long hours and critical decisions.

      ▲ *Statistic*: Surgeons who practice mindfulness report 25% lower stress levels, according to a 2021 study in *The American Journal of Surgery*.

Actionable Insights:

* **Pre-Surgery Ritual**: Spend 2 minutes visualizing the surgery, focusing on each step. Pair this with slow, deliberate breaths.

* **Post-Surgery Reflection**: Spend 5 minutes reflecting on the procedure—what went well, what could improve—without self-criticism.

Simple Mindfulness Techniques for Surgeons

1. **Breathing Exercises:**

   ❖ Practice *box breathing*: Inhale for 4 seconds, hold for 4 seconds, exhale for 4 seconds, and hold again for 4 seconds. This method calms the nervous system and sharpens focus.

2. **Body Scans:**

   ❖ Perform a quick body scan during breaks. Notice areas of tension and consciously relax them.

3. **Mindful Eating:**

   ❖ Pay attention to the taste, texture, and aroma of your food during breaks. This fosters a sense of presence and enjoyment.

4. **Gratitude Practice:**

   ❖ At the end of each day, write down three things you're grateful for, such as a successful surgery or a patient's thank-you note, helpful mentors or collegues.

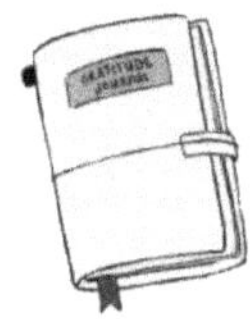

Interactive Element:

Guided Practice:

✳   Close your eyes and take a deep breath. As you exhale, silently say, "I am calm and relaxed." Repeat this five times, noticing how your body feels.

Challenges in Practicing Mindfulness and How to Overcome Them

1.   **Lack of Time:**

    ◆   As a surgeon, free time is scarce. However, mindfulness doesn't require long sessions. A few minutes a day can make a difference.

        ⅄   *Tip*: Integrate mindfulness into existing routines, like washing hands before surgery or during your commute.

2.   **Difficulty Staying Present:**

    ◆   The mind naturally wanders, especially during stressful moments. Practice gently bringing your focus back without frustration.

       ▲   *Tip*: Use a mantra like "Focus on now" for 5 times when distractions arise.

3.   **Skepticism About Benefits:**

     ◆   Some may view mindfulness as abstract or unscientific. Rely on research-based evidence to overcome doubts.

       ▲   *Example*: Share stories of colleagues who use mindfulness to enhance their performance and well-being.

Interactive Element:

Question:

✳   "What are your biggest barriers to practicing mindfulness? How could you address them in small, manageable steps?"

Actionable Takeaway:

Start with just 1 minute of mindful breathing each day. Build this habit gradually, and observe how it transforms your focus and emotional resilience. Remember, mindfulness is not about perfection but about progress.

This chapter not only educates readers on mindfulness but also empowers them to take actionable steps, supported by evidence and interactive elements, to enhance their well-being and performance as surgeons.

Recap and Summary

Key Points Recap:

1.   Mindfulness involves cultivating awareness, acceptance, and non-judgment, helping surgeons manage stress and improve performance.

2. Scientific research shows that mindfulness enhances focus, emotional regulation, and overall well-being.

3. For surgeons, mindfulness offers benefits like improved attention, reduced stress, and better patient interactions.

4. Simple practices like breathing exercises, body scans, and gratitude journaling can make mindfulness accessible.

5. Overcoming barriers such as time constraints and skepticism is crucial for integrating mindfulness into daily life.

3

Practical Mindfulness Techniques for Surgeons

Introduction

For surgeons, the demands of the operating room require split-second decision-making, unwavering focus, and emotional control. However, the high-pressure environment can lead to stress, burnout, and fatigue. Integrating mindfulness techniques into your daily routine can help improve focus, emotional resilience, and patient outcomes. This chapter provides practical, evidence-based strategies that fit seamlessly into a surgeon's demanding schedule, offering tools to remain calm and present, even in the most high-stress situations.

Mindfulness Techniques Tailored to a Surgeon's Schedule

1. **Breathing Exercises for Instant Calm**

   ◆ **Box Breathing:**

     ⋏ Inhale for 4 seconds, hold for 4 seconds, exhale for 4 seconds, and hold for another 4 seconds.

     ⋏ *Why it works:* Activates the parasympathetic nervous system, reducing stress.

- ◆ **Alternate Nostril Breathing:**

  - ⋏ Use your thumb to close your right nostril, inhale through the left nostril, close the left nostril, and exhale through the right nostril.

  - ⋏ *Application*: Before starting rounds, this technique helps center your mind.

2. **Guided Meditation for Surgeons on the Go**

   - ◆ Use apps like Headspace or Insight Timer for 5-minute guided meditations during coffee breaks or while commuting.

   - ◆ Focused meditations for surgeons might include themes like grounding before surgery or recovering from stressful cases.

3. **Micro Mindfulness Techniques**

   - ◆ **Handwashing Practice:**

     - ⋏ During the scrubbing process before surgery, pay attention to the sensations of water and soap on your hands. This ritual can serve as a mindfulness anchor.

   - ◆ **Mindful Walking:**

     - ⋏ Walk mindfully down hospital corridors by focusing on your steps, breath, and surroundings.

Actionable Insight:

✱ Start with one of these techniques and gradually incorporate more into your daily routine. Consistency is key.

Mindfulness in Preoperative and Postoperative Settings

1. **Preoperative Mindfulness**

   - ◆ **Visualization Techniques:**

     - ⋏ Before surgery, visualize the steps of the procedure, focusing on a successful outcome.

     - ⋏ Grounding Exercises:

      A Practice grounding techniques such as feeling your feet on the floor and focusing on your breath for 2 minutes before entering the OR.

  • **Setting Intentions**:

      A Take a moment to set an intention for the surgery, such as, "I will remain calm and focused throughout this procedure."

2. **Postoperative Reflection**

  • **Debrief with Mindfulness**:

      A After the surgery, spend 5 minutes reflecting on the procedure without judgment. Focus on what went well and identify areas for improvement.

      A *Tip*: Use a journal to record these reflections.

  • **Body Scan for Recovery**:

      A Perform a quick body scan to release tension accumulated during the surgery. Start from your head and move down to your toes, consciously relaxing each area.

Actionable Insight:

* Schedule 5 minutes before and after each surgery to practice preoperative and postoperative mindfulness techniques.

Real-Time Strategies for Staying Present in High-Stress Moments

1. **The STOP Technique**

  • **Steps**:

      A *S*: Stop what you are doing.

      A *T*: Take a deep breath.

- ⮤ *O*: Observe your thoughts, feelings, and surroundings.

- ⮤ *P*: Proceed with awareness and focus.

- ⮤ *Example*: During a sudden complication in surgery, using the STOP technique can help regain composure and think clearly.

2. **3-Second Breathing Pause**

   - ◆ Take a single deep breath in and out to center yourself before responding to a stressful situation.

   - ◆ *Scenario*: A nurse informs you of a critical patient issue mid-surgery. This pause allows you to respond thoughtfully rather than react impulsively.

3. **Labeling Emotions**

   - ◆ Identify and label the emotions you are feeling in the moment.

   - ◆ *Example*: "I'm feeling anxious because this case is complex." This practice creates a sense of control and reduces the intensity of negative emotions.

4. **Mindful Listening in Team Communication**

   - ◆ Focus on listening fully to your team members without interrupting or formulating a response prematurely.

Actionable Insight:

✳ Practice these real-time strategies during the next stressful moment and observe how they improve your response.

Suggested Resources:

✳ **Books:**

   - ◆ *The SILVA MINDS CONTROL METHOD by Jose silva*

   - ◆ *MINDSET by DR CAROL S.DECK*

◆ *Marcus aurelius* MEDITATIONS

Overcoming Barriers to Practicing Mindfulness in Surgery

1. **Limited Time**

    ◆ **Solution**: Integrate micro-mindfulness techniques into existing routines, such as handwashing or walking to the OR.

2. **Doubts About Effectiveness**

    ◆ **Solution**: Start with small, tangible practices and track their impact on stress and focus.

3. **Perception of Mindfulness as "Soft"**

    ◆ **Solution**: Share scientific evidence and real-life examples to highlight its impact on performance and well-being.

Interactive Element:

✳ Reflect on this question: "What small change could you make in your current routine to incorporate mindfulness?"

Recap and Summary

Mindfulness is not about achieving perfection but about cultivating presence and resilience. By integrating these techniques into your daily routine, you can improve not only your performance but also your overall well-being as a surgeon.

This detailed chapter provides actionable strategies, evidence, and real-life examples to help surgeons adopt mindfulness in their demanding practice.

Key Takeaways:

1. Mindfulness techniques such as breathing exercises, body scans, and visualization can fit seamlessly into a surgeon's schedule.

2. Preoperative and postoperative mindfulness enhance focus, reduce stress, and support emotional recovery.

3. Real-time strategies like the STOP technique and mindful listening help surgeons stay present during high-stress situations.

4. Case studies demonstrate the transformative impact of mindfulness on both individual surgeons and surgical teams.

Managing Stress in the OR and Beyond

Introduction: The Pressure Cooker of Surgery

Picture this: You're in the OR, the patient's blood pressure drops, alarms beep, and all eyes turn to you for a decision. Being a surgeon is often like playing a high-stakes chess match on a rollercoaster—intense, unpredictable, and exhausting. Stress is part of the job, but chronic stress can lead to burnout, impaired decision-making, and even health problems.

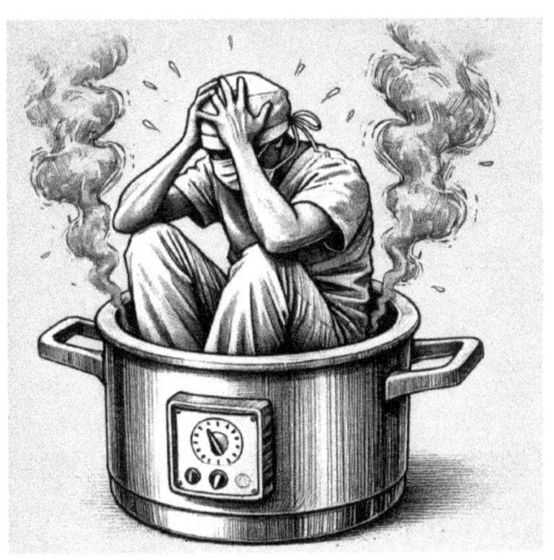

This chapter will explore how to recognize stress, practical strategies to manage it in the moment, and long-term habits for resilience. Let's dive in with a healthy mix of science, actionable tips, and a bit of humor (because laughter is great medicine, too!).

Recognizing the Signs and Symptoms of Stress

Acute vs. Chronic Stress

✳ **Acute Stress**: Sudden, short-lived, and often tied to emergencies (e.g., handling unexpected complications in surgery).

  ◆ *Symptoms*: Rapid heartbeat, sweating, tunnel vision, irritability, or a racing mind.

✳ **Chronic Stress**: Long-term, accumulates over time due to constant pressure.

  ◆ *Symptoms*: Fatigue, insomnia, reduced focus, emotional detachment, or even physical symptoms like headaches and back pain.

Why Recognizing Stress Matters

✳ Ignoring stress is like ignoring a ticking time bomb. Recognizing it early allows you to respond effectively before it impacts your health or performance.

Interactive Element:

✳ Ask yourself: "When was the last time I felt overwhelmed at work? What were the physical or emotional signs?" Write down your observations.

....

....

Coping with Stress in High-Stakes Environments

1. **The Power of Breathing**

  ◆ **Technique**: 4-7-8 Breathing

    ⅄ Inhale for 4 seconds, hold for 7 seconds, exhale for 8 seconds.

> ▲ *Why it works:* Slows your heart rate and engages the parasympathetic nervous system.

> ▲ *In the* OR: Use this technique during a momentary pause, like waiting for test results or while scrubbing in.

2. **Visualization Techniques**

   ◆ Picture a calm, successful outcome. Visualize yourself confidently managing the procedure.

3. **Humor as a Stress Reliever**

   ◆ Share a light joke (appropriate, of course) with your team to break tension.

   As the surgery stretched into its fifth hour with fatigue setting in, the surgeon looked up and said, "If anyone's thinking about what's for dinner, let me remind you—this guy's stomach is not on the menu." The room erupted in quiet laughter, and the team's mood lightened, helping them push through the remainder of the procedure with renewed focus.

4. **Quick Grounding Techniques**

   ◆ Focus on physical sensations like your feet on the floor or the feel of your gloves.

Interactive Element:

✱ During your next procedure, try a quick grounding technique and reflect afterward: Did it help you focus or calm down?

Long-Term Resilience-Building Habits

1. **Reflective Journaling**

   ◆ Spend 5–10 minutes after your shift writing about your day. Reflect on what went well, what didn't, and what you learned.

    ▲   *Benefits*: Improves self-awareness, reduces mental clutter, and fosters growth.

2. **Mindfulness-Based Stress Reduction (MBSR)**

   ◆ A structured program combining meditation, body scans, and yoga to reduce stress.

       ▲ *Evidence*: A study in *JAMA Surgery* found that surgeons who practiced MBSR reported 25% lower stress levels and better emotional resilience.

   ◆ *Resources*:

       ▲ Book: *Full Catastrophe Living* by Jon Kabat-Zinn

       ▲ App: *Calm*

3. **Exercise and Physical Health**

   ◆ Even 30 minutes of moderate exercise (e.g., walking, swimming) can boost endorphins and reduce stress.

   ◆ If surgeons can stand for hours in the OR, surely you can find 30 minutes to walk—just think of it as another procedure, but for your heart!

4. **Building a Support Network**

   ◆ Talk to colleagues, mentors, or a therapist. Sharing your struggles doesn't make you weak; it makes you human.

Interactive Element:

✱ Write down one small change you can make this week to build resilience (e.g., start journaling, try a new workout, or practice a 5-minute meditation).

....

....

Stress is inevitable in surgery, but it doesn't have to control you. By integrating these strategies into your routine, you can stay sharp, balanced, and, dare we say, even enjoy the ride. After all, managing stress is like suturing—precise, deliberate, and deeply satisfying when done right.

Recap and Summary

Key Takeaways:

1. Recognizing stress is the first step to managing it effectively.

2. Acute stress can be managed with techniques like breathing exercises, visualization, and humor.

3. Long-term habits, including journaling, mindfulness, and exercise, build resilience against chronic stress.

4. Laughter isn't just fun—it's a powerful stress reliever.

5

Building Emotional Resilience

Introduction: Emotional Resilience – The Unsung Hero of Surgery

Surgery isn't just about scalpels and sutures; it's a profession that tests the limits of human endurance—emotionally, mentally, and physically. Emotional resilience is the secret sauce that allows surgeons to navigate the highs and lows of this demanding field. Without it, challenging cases can lead to frustration, exhaustion, and, ultimately, burnout.

In this chapter, we'll explore the concept of emotional resilience, why it's crucial for surgeons, tools to manage emotions, and methods to develop compassion without burning out. We'll also lighten the mood with humor and interactive sessions because, let's face it, even surgeons need a good laugh.

What is Emotional Resilience, and Why Does It Matter?

Defining Emotional Resilience

* The ability to adapt to stress, recover from setbacks, and maintain emotional balance in challenging situations.

* *Analogy*: Emotional resilience is like your surgical instruments—if they're not sharp and well-maintained, you're in for a rough time.

Importance in Surgery

* Surgeons encounter emotional triggers daily: patient outcomes, family interactions, and their own self-doubt.

* Resilience helps you stay calm, make sound decisions, and avoid emotional exhaustion.

Interactive Session

* Reflect on a time you faced an emotionally taxing situation in surgery. What helped you bounce back? Write down three strategies you used (or wish you had).

Tools for Managing Emotions During Challenging Cases

1. **The STOP Technique**

   ◆ **S**top: Pause for a moment.

   ◆ **T**ake a deep breath.

   ◆ **O**bserve: Identify your emotions without judgment.

   ◆ **P**roceed: Respond calmly and thoughtfully.

2. **Naming Emotions**

   ◆ Labeling feelings like fear, anger, or sadness reduces their intensity.

   ◆ Studies show naming emotions activates the brain's rational centers, reducing emotional overwhelm.

3. **Cognitive Reframing**

   ◆ Shift your perspective: Instead of "I failed this surgery," think, "I learned what not to do next time."

Interactive Element

* Think of a recent emotional challenge. Write down the emotion you felt, then reframe the situation positively.

Developing Compassion and Empathy Without Burnout

1. **Setting Emotional Boundaries**

   ◆ Compassion doesn't mean absorbing every patient's pain. Set boundaries to protect your mental health.

   ◆ Visualize a shield around you that lets empathy in but keeps overwhelming emotions out.

2. **Practicing Empathetic Communication**

   ◆ Listen actively and acknowledge patients 'feelings.

      ▲ *Example:* Instead of saying, "It's a minor complication," try, "I understand this is concerning. Let me explain how we'll address it."

3. **Self-Compassion**

   ◆ Treat yourself as you would a colleague in the same situation.

   ◆ Self-compassion reduces stress and promotes resilience in high-stakes professions.

4. **Mindfulness and Compassion Meditation**

   ◆ Guided meditations focusing on compassion can enhance empathy without draining you emotionally.

Building Emotional Resilience Over Time

1. **Reflective Journaling**

   ◆ Write about challenging cases to process emotions and identify growth opportunities.

      ▲ *Example:* After a failed surgery, Dr. M journaled her thoughts, helping his process guilt and find areas for improvement.

2. **Peer Support Groups**

   ◆ Discussing experiences with colleagues normalizes emotional struggles and fosters resilience.

   ◆ Create a monthly meet-up with fellow residents or surgeons to share stories and strategies.

3. **Gratitude Practice**

   ◆ Focus on what went well each day, no matter how small.

      ⋏ *Example*: I am greatful to my PATIENT for giving me oppurtunity to treat him, so that I am learning from them.

4. **Humor as a Daily Habit**

   ◆ Start meetings with a funny anecdote or share humorous but appropriate OR moments with your team.

Summary Key Points

1. Emotional resilience is critical for navigating the emotional and mental challenges of surgery.

2. Recognizing and naming emotions can reduce their intensity and prevent overwhelm.

3. Techniques like the STOP method and cognitive reframing are powerful tools for managing emotions in high-stress situations.

4. Humor is an underrated yet effective way to relieve stress and foster connection in the OR.

5. Compassionate communication enhances patient relationships but requires emotional boundaries to prevent burnout.

6. Self-compassion is just as important as compassion for others— treat yourself with kindness after setbacks.

7. Reflective journaling and gratitude practices build long-term emotional strength.

8. Peer support groups normalize emotional struggles and create a sense of camaraderie.

9. Combining mindfulness with compassion reduces emotional exhaustion while increasing empathy.

10. Resilience isn't a solo journey—teams that practice emotional resilience together thrive together.

6

Maintaining Physical and Mental Health

Introduction: The Foundation of a Surgeon's Success

Surgery is often likened to running a marathon that never ends. Surgeons push their physical and mental limits daily, often sacrificing their own health in the process. However, the truth is clear: a healthy surgeon is a better surgeon. Physical fitness enhances stamina and focus, while mental well-being ensures resilience, patience, and empathy.

This chapter explores why physical and mental health are critical for surgeons, offering actionable strategies to fit wellness into a busy schedule. We'll cover fitness, nutrition, sleep hygiene, and mental health practices like therapy and self-care. Expect practical tips, a touch of humor, and interactive elements to inspire you to prioritize your well-being.

The Role of Physical Fitness in Surgical Excellence

1. **Why Physical Fitness Matters**

    ◆ **Stamina and Endurance**: Long hours in the OR require physical strength to prevent fatigue and maintain precision.

    ◆ **Mental Clarity**: Exercise improves cognitive functions like focus, memory, and problem-solving.

◆ **Stress Relief**: Physical activity reduces cortisol levels, combating chronic stress.

2. **Quick Fitness Strategies for Busy Schedules**

    ◆ **The 10-Minute Workout**: High-intensity interval training (HIIT) sessions that can be done at home.

        ▲ *Example*: 30 seconds each of squats, push-ups, planks, and burpees, repeated three times.

    ◆ **Staircase Cardio**: Opt for stairs instead of elevators during rounds.

    ◆ **Yoga for Surgeons**: Simple poses to stretch your back, neck, and shoulders after hours of surgery.

    ◆ *Pose Recommendation*: The "Surgeon's Savior Stretch" (Child's Pose with extended arms).

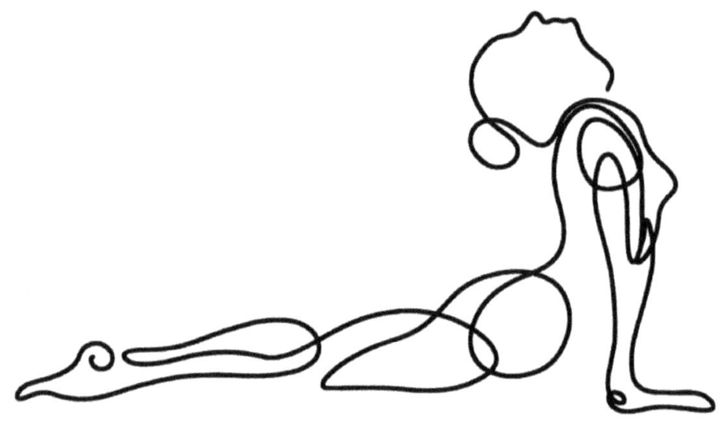

Interactive Element

✱ Challenge: Set a timer for 10 minutes and do a mini-workout. Log how you feel afterward—more alert? Less stressed?

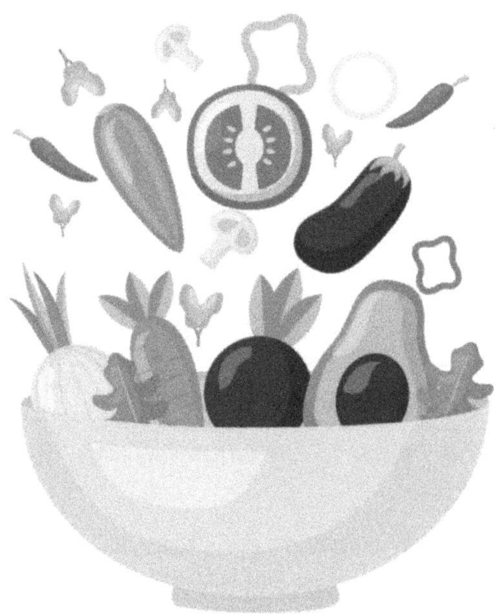

Nutrition as a Power Source

1. **Fueling Your Body for Performance**

   ◆ **Balanced Diet Principles:**

      ▲ Protein for muscle repair (e.g., eggs, lean meat, lentils).

      ▲ Complex carbs for sustained energy (e.g., whole grains, sweet potatoes).

      ▲ Healthy fats for brain function (e.g., nuts, seeds, avocado).

      ▲ Hydration for focus and stamina.

      ▲ "Fast food may be quick, but so is burnout. Choose wisely!"

Sleep Hygiene for Surgeons

1. **Why Sleep is Crucial**

    ◆   **Performance Enhancement**: Sleep improves reaction time, memory, and decision-making—all vital in surgery.

    ◆   **Burnout Prevention**: Lack of sleep contributes to irritability and emotional exhaustion.

    ◆   **Immune Support**: Rest boosts your body's ability to fight infections.

2. **Strategies for Better Sleep**

    ◆   **Power Naps**: 15–20 minutes during breaks can improve alertness.

    ◆   **Sleep Environment**: Use blackout curtains, white noise, and a cool room for optimal sleep.

    ◆   **Wind-Down Routine**: Avoid screens for an hour before bed; try reading or meditating instead.

Interactive Element

*   Create a "sleep checklist" of habits you can adopt this week. Track your hours and note how you feel each morning.

Mental Health Maintenance

1. **Recognizing Mental Health as a Priority**

    ◆   Mental health impacts your ability to manage stress, connect with patients, and make sound decisions.

2. **Therapy and Peer Support**

    ◆   **Professional Help**: Therapy isn't just for crises; it's a tool for self-awareness and growth.

        ⋏   *Resource*: Cognitive Behavioral Therapy (CBT) for managing stress and anxiety.

◆ **Peer Support Groups**: Sharing challenges with fellow surgeons reduces feelings of isolation.

3. **Self-Care Practices**

◆ **Mindfulness Meditation**: 5-minute breathing exercises to reset your mind.

▴ *Exercise*: Close your eyes and focus on your breath for 10 cycles. Notice the calm.

◆ **Hobbies for Relaxation**: Pursue non-medical interests to recharge emotionally.

▴ Examples: Painting, gardening, playing a musical instrument, listening to music.

Interactive Element

* Write down one mental health habit you'll start today. Share it with a trusted friend or colleague.

....

....

Combining Physical and Mental Wellness into a Routine

1. **The Synergy Between Body and Mind**

◆ Physical health fuels mental clarity; mental health drives physical motivation.

◆ A well-rested surgeon is less likely to skip their morning workout, creating a positive feedback loop.

2. **Building a Sustainable Routine**

◆ **Morning Rituals**: 10-minute mindfulness practice + quick workout.

- ◆ **Daily Gratitude**: Write one thing you're thankful for each day.

- ◆ **Evening Reflections**: Journal lessons learned and goals for tomorrow.

"Maintaining physical and mental health as a surgeon isn't easy, but remember: you're the best advocate for your own health. And if anyone complains about your wellness breaks, just tell them it's doctor's orders!"

This chapter empowers surgeons to view self-care not as a luxury, but as an essential part of their journey to excellence, both in the OR and beyond.

Summary: Key Takeaways for Wellness

1. Physical fitness enhances stamina and mental clarity, essential for long surgeries.

2. Short, high-intensity workouts are perfect for busy surgeons.

3. Nutrition is fuel: prioritise protein, complex carbs, and hydration.

4. Meal prep saves time and ensures balanced eating.

5. Quality sleep improves decision-making and reduces burnout.

6. Create a calming sleep environment with routines like meditation.

7. Mental health deserves the same attention as physical health.

8. Therapy and peer support normalise challenges and provide relief.

9. Hobbies and mindfulness exercises recharge your emotional reserves.

10. Integrate wellness habits into a routine for long-term benefits.

7

Balancing Professional and Personal Life

Introduction: The Tightrope Walk of a Surgeon's Life

Surgeons are often caught between two worlds: the high-pressure demands of their profession and the equally important need for personal fulfilment. Achieving balance feels like walking a tightrope over an abyss of burnout. But here's the good news—work-life balance is not a myth; it's a skill.

This chapter explores the art of balancing a demanding surgical career with a fulfilling personal life. We'll discuss setting boundaries, practical time management, and how mindfulness can help reduce guilt while staying present in personal moments. Expect humor, relatable anecdotes, and actionable strategies to bring harmony to your dual roles.

What Does Work-Life Balance Look Like for Surgeons?

1. **Redefining Work-Life Balance**

    ◆ Work-life balance isn't about splitting time equally; it's about ensuring that both professional and personal priorities are met over time.

◆ Think of it as a pendulum: sometimes it swings toward work, other times toward life, but it should never stay stuck in one direction.

2. **Why Boundaries Matter**

◆ Setting clear boundaries protects your mental and physical health.

    ▲ Example: Defining "on-call" time versus "personal time" ensures you don't feel perpetually available.

◆ Boundaries also preserve relationships by communicating when and how you're present.

◆ Ask yourself: *What does balance mean for me?* Write down three personal priorities and three professional priorities.

1. ....

2. ....

3. ....

4. ....

5. ....

6. ....

8

Scheduling Personal Time, Family Time, and Rest

1. **Practical Scheduling Tips**

   ◆ **Block Time for Personal Commitments**: Treat your family dinner or gym session like a surgery—non-negotiable.

     ▲ *Example*: Schedule one "date night" or family game night each week.

   ◆ **Plan Downtime Proactively**: Use calendar apps to block rest days and stick to them.

   ◆ **The Power of Micro-Moments**:

   ◆ Use 5-minute breaks to call a loved one or practice a mindfulness exercise.

2. **Delegating and Saying No**

   ◆ Recognise when to delegate tasks at work to protect your personal time.

     ▲ Example: Let a junior resident handle routine paperwork while you take 15 minutes to recharge.

   ◆ Learn the power of saying no: "I can't take on this additional case today, but I can tomorrow."

- Create a "Personal Priority Chart" for the week. Highlight time for family, hobbies, and rest, then schedule work tasks around it.

Using Mindfulness to Stay Present

1. **The Guilt Factor**

   - Many surgeons feel guilty for taking personal time, fearing it compromises their professional responsibilities.

   - Reality Check: You can't pour from an empty cup. Personal time enhances professional performance.

2. **How Mindfulness Helps**

   - Mindfulness reduces feelings of guilt by anchoring you in the present.

   - When with family, focus on the conversation, not the patient list.

   - At work, give your full attention to the task at hand, knowing you've scheduled personal time later.

3. **Simple Mindfulness Exercises**

   - **Before Switching Roles**: Take three deep breaths and visualise stepping into your next role (e.g., from surgeon to parent or friend).

   - **Gratitude Journaling**: At the end of the day, write down three things you're grateful for in your professional and personal life.

Interactive Element

✳ Practice a "Transition Ritual." After work, take 5 minutes to breathe deeply, stretch, or listen to a calming song before engaging with your family or hobbies.

Real-Life Strategies for Work-Life Balance

Handling Unexpected Demands

✳   **Flexibility Without Guilt**: It's okay if emergencies occasionally disrupt your personal plans.

✳   Mindset Shift: Focus on how you can adjust future schedules to compensate.

✳   **Communicate Transparently**: Let your family or friends know about unpredictable work demands while reaffirming your commitment to them.

Interactive Element

✳   Reflect on a time when work disrupted your personal plans. What could you do differently next time? Write down your strategies.

....

....

Long-Term Strategies for Sustainable Balance

1.   Make Balance a Habit

◆   Incorporate routines that reinforce both professional and personal priorities:

➤   *Morning*: Start with a mindfulness exercise to set the tone for the day.

➤   *Evening*: Dedicate time to a hobby, even if it is 15 minutes.

2.   Celebrate Small Wins

◆   Acknowledge moments when you successfully balanced both worlds.

➤   Example: "I completed two surgeries today and still made it to my kid's soccer game!"

3. **Evaluate and Adjust Regularly**

    ◆ Weekly, monthly, quarterly Review: Assess your work-life balance and make adjustments as needed.

Interactive Element

* Create a "Balance Journal." Record one professional achievement and one personal joy each day. At the end of the week, reflect on how balanced your life feels.

Work-life balance is like surgery: it requires precision, planning, and adaptability. While the demands of your career may be intense, remember that prioritising personal time isn't selfish—it's essential. After all, a balanced surgeon is a better surgeon. And who knows? You might even find time to perfect your golf swing—or your burnt toast recovery skills.

Summary: Key Takeaways for Work-Life Balance

1. Work-life balance isn't perfection; it's about prioritisation over time.

2. Set clear boundaries to protect your mental and physical health.

3. Schedule personal time as firmly as professional commitments.

4. Use mindfulness to reduce guilt and stay present in each role.

5. Take advantage of micro-moments to connect with loved ones or recharge.

6. Learn to say no and delegate when necessary.

7. Evaluate your balance regularly and adjust as needed.

8. Celebrate small wins—progress is better than perfection.

9

Patient Interaction with Mindfulness and Empathy

Introduction: The Art of Human Connection in Surgery

A surgeon's skill is often measured by the precision of their scalpel, but the true essence of patient care lies beyond the operating room. It's in the words you choose, the compassion you show, and the way you connect with patients and their families.

This chapter focuses on using mindfulness and empathy to improve patient interactions, tackle difficult conversations, and maintain emotional balance in challenging situations. From techniques to enhance bedside manner to practical tips for managing intense emotions, you'll learn how to build trust, provide comfort, and leave a lasting positive impact.

Let's explore the softer side of surgery—where science meets humanity. And don't worry, we'll keep it light-hearted where we can, because patient interactions aren't always serious (just ask the patient who thought "general surgeon" meant you were in the army).

The Foundations of Mindful Patient Interaction

1. **Why Mindfulness Matters in Patient Communication**

   ◆ **Being Fully Present:** Patients can sense when your mind is elsewhere. Mindfulness helps you focus entirely on the patient in front of you.

- ◆ **Improved Listening**: Active listening fosters trust and ensures you don't miss critical information.

- ◆ **Reduced Stress for Both Parties**: A calm, mindful approach reassures anxious patients and creates a sense of safety.

2. **Key Principles of Mindful Communication**

- ◆ **Pause Before You Speak**: Take a deep breath before responding to challenging questions or emotions.

- ◆ **Reflect Empathy in Your Words**: Use phrases like, "I understand this is difficult for you," to validate their feelings.

- ◆ **Body Language Counts**: Maintain eye contact, nod occasionally, and avoid distractions like checking your phone.

- ◆ "When a patient says, 'I just Googled my symptoms,' mindfulness is the only thing stopping you from replying, 'And did Google suggest surgery too?'"

Techniques for Compassionate Communication

1. **The Power of Empathy**

- ◆ Empathy doesn't mean agreeing with a patient; it means understanding their perspective.

  - ⋏ Example: A patient might refuse surgery due to fear. Empathy helps you address the fear rather than dismissing it.

2. **Practical Communication Techniques**

- ◆ **Teach-Back Method**: After explaining a procedure or diagnosis, ask the patient to repeat it in their own words to ensure understanding.

- ◆ **Use Simple Language**: Replace medical jargon with relatable terms.

  - ⋏ Instead of "You have a laceration," say, "You have a deep cut that needs stitches."

◆ **Acknowledge Emotions**: "It's natural to feel nervous about this procedure."

3. **Dealing with Emotional Situations**

   ◆ **Breaking Bad News**:

      ▲ Be direct yet compassionate: "I'm sorry to share this news, but…"

      ▲ Allow silence; patients may need time to process.

   ◆ **Handling Anger or Frustration**:

      ▲ Stay calm and validate their feelings: "I hear that this is upsetting for you."

Strategies for Handling Difficult Patient Interactions

1. **Recognizing Emotional Triggers**

   ◆ Identify moments that challenge your patience or empathy, such as:

      ▲ A demanding patient asking repetitive questions.

      ▲ A family member questioning your expertise.

2. **Mindfulness Techniques for Difficult Situations**

   ◆ **Deep Breathing**: Take 3–5 deep breaths to ground yourself before responding.

   ◆ **Name the Emotion**: Internally acknowledge your feelings (e.g., "I'm feeling frustrated") to regain control.

   ◆ **Mantras for Calmness**: Use phrases like, "This is not personal; this is about the patient's fear."

3. **Setting Boundaries**

   ◆ It's okay to redirect conversations when necessary:

      ▲ "I understand your concerns, but let's focus on the next steps for your care."

♦ "Sometimes, being a surgeon means listening to a patient describe their unrelated knee pain during a consult about appendicitis—and nodding like it's the most relevant thing in the world."

Incorporating Mindfulness and Empathy at the Bedside

1. **The Role of Empathy in Bedside Manner**

   ♦ Patients remember how you made them feel more than what you said. A kind tone and a compassionate smile can ease fear.

2. **Mindfulness During Patient Counselling**

   ♦ **Focus on the Now**: Instead of worrying about the next patient or procedure, devote your full attention to the current conversation.

   ♦ **Mindful Touch**: A reassuring hand on the shoulder (if appropriate) can convey more comfort than words.

3. **Handling Family Dynamics Mindfully**

   ♦ Family members often have high emotions. Address their concerns with calmness and clarity:

      ⋏ "I understand you're worried. Here's what we're doing to care for your loved one."

Interactive element

✳ During your next patient interaction, consciously practice one new mindfulness or empathy technique. Reflect afterward on how it felt for both you and the patient.

....

Building Long-Term Relationships with Patients

1. **Trust is Built Over Time**

   ♦ Consistent, empathetic communication fosters trust, even during complex treatments.

2. **Balancing Professionalism and Warmth**

    ◆ Find the sweet spot between being approachable and maintaining authority. Patients appreciate warmth but expect expertise.

The Value of Consistency

✳ Habit of visiting each post-op patient daily, even for a brief check-in. Patients frequently praised her for making them feel valued, contributing to higher patient satisfaction scores.

✳ "Building trust with patients is easy: just don't accidentally say 'Oops' during surgery."

Patient interactions are as much about the heart as they are about the brain. By integrating mindfulness and empathy, you can turn even the most challenging conversations into opportunities to comfort, heal, and build trust. Remember, the scalpel may fix the body, but your words and presence heal the soul—and sometimes, that's what patients remember the most.

Summary: Key Takeaways for Mindful and Empathetic Patient Interactions

1. Mindfulness helps you stay present and focused during patient interactions.

2. Empathy fosters trust, even in difficult or emotional situations.

3. Use clear, simple language to ensure understanding.

4. Acknowledge patient emotions and validate their concerns.

5. Employ mindfulness techniques like deep breathing to stay calm in challenging moments.

6. Set boundaries to guide conversations effectively without losing compassion.

7. Consistent, empathetic communication builds lasting trust and satisfaction.

8. Humor, when appropriate, can diffuse tension and connect on a human level.

10

Building a Support System in Residency

Introduction: No Surgeon is an Island

Residency is often described as a solo marathon. The long hours, emotional rollercoasters, and the relentless learning curve can make it feel isolating. But here's the secret: no one actually gets through it alone. Behind every successful surgeon is a network of mentors, colleagues, family, and friends who provide encouragement, guidance, and the occasional reality check (like reminding you to eat something other than hospital vending machine snacks).

This chapter is about the power of connection. A strong support system isn't just a nice-to-have—it's essential for surviving and thriving in residency. From mentors who guide you to friends who let you vent, we'll explore how to build and sustain these vital relationships.

The Role of Mentors in Residency

1. **Why Mentors Matter**

   ◆ **Guidance in Chaos**: Mentors provide clarity during challenging moments, from career decisions to managing tough cases.

◆ **Role Models**: They show you what kind of surgeon—and person—you aspire to be.

◆ **Emotional Anchor**: A good mentor can offer perspective and reassurance when the going gets tough.

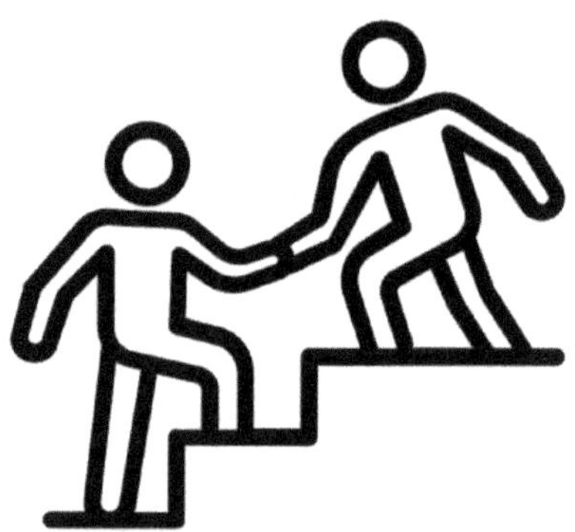

2. **Finding the Right Mentor**

◆ **Shared Values**: Look for someone whose approach to medicine aligns with yours.

◆ **Availability**: A mentor should have time to genuinely invest in your growth.

◆ **Trust and Respect**: This relationship works best when it's built on mutual trust.

◆ "A mentor is like a GPS—they guide you in the right direction, but they can't stop you from taking a wrong turn (or missing rounds)."

Leaning on Colleagues and Peers

1. **Shared Experiences, Shared Strength**

◆ Your co-residents are the only ones who truly understand what you're going through—they're in the trenches with you.

◆ **Venting Without Judgment**: A quick venting session about a difficult case can lighten your mental load.

2. **Building Camaraderie**

   ◆ **Support, Not Competition**: While surgical training is competitive, it's essential to see your peers as allies.

   ◆ **Celebrating Successes Together**: From nailing a tough procedure to completing a gruelling rotation, small celebrations can boost morale.

Interactive Element

✳ Organize a "win of the week" session with your peers where you each share a small victory or positive moment from the week.

The Role of Family and Friends

1. **Family as Emotional Anchors**

   ◆ Family members provide unconditional love and a safe space to decompress.

   ◆ **Maintaining Connections**: Even a quick call home can bring perspective and comfort.

2. **Balancing Residency and Relationships**

   ◆ **Scheduling Time**: Plan regular phone calls or meet-ups to keep your relationships strong.

   ◆ **Communicating Your Needs**: Be honest about your time constraints but also make an effort to stay connected.

3. **Friends Outside Medicine**

   ◆ Non-medical friends can offer a refreshing perspective and remind you there's life beyond the hospital.

   ◆ They're also more likely to laugh at your jokes that don't involve anatomy or surgery puns.

   ◆ Schedule a "social recharge" activity this week, whether it's a quick call to a friend or dinner with a loved one. Notice how it impacts your mood.

Asking for Help Without Hesitation

Breaking the Stigma

* Many residents hesitate to ask for help, fearing it shows weakness. In reality, it's a sign of strength.

* **Recognising When You Need Support**:

  ◆ Feeling overwhelmed or burnt out? It's time to reach out.

* Write down one resource or person you could reach out to for support in a challenging moment.

* "Asking for help isn't weakness—it's like calling in a consult. Even superheroes need a sidekick."

Nurturing Your Support System

1. **Investing in Relationships**

   ◆ Relationships require effort. Regular check-ins, small gestures, and expressions of gratitude go a long way.

2. **Letting Go of Toxic Connections**

   ◆ Not all relationships are beneficial. It's okay to distance yourself from negative influences that drain your energy.

Interactive Element

* Send a thank-you note or message to someone in your support system this week.

* "Remember, a great support system is like a Wi-Fi connection— strong, reliable, and there when you need it most."

In the high-pressure world of residency, your support system isn't just a safety net—it's your lifeline. Whether it's a mentor's wise words, a friend's laughter, or a colleague's solidarity, these connections remind you that you're never truly alone. So, invest in them, nurture them, and let them be the wind beneath your (scrub-covered) wings.

Summary:Key Takeaways for Building a Support System in Residency

1. Mentors provide guidance, reassurance, and inspiration—seek them out.

2. Co-residents understand your struggles like no one else; lean on them for support.

3. Family and friends offer grounding and a reminder of life outside medicine.

4. Non-medical friends can refresh your perspective and keep things light.

5. Asking for help isn't weakness; it's a strength and a step toward resilience.

6. Use available resources like counselling, support groups, and online communities.

7. Invest in your relationships by showing appreciation and staying connected.

8. Let go of toxic relationships that drain your emotional reserves.

11

Cultivating Hobbies and Interests Outside Medicine

Introduction: More Than Just a Surgeon

As a surgical resident, your identity can feel inextricably tied to your white coat, stethoscope, and the OR. But beneath the scrubs is a multifaceted individual with passions, dreams, and interests that extend far beyond medicine. Cultivating hobbies isn't just about fun—it's about preserving your mental well-being, fostering creativity, and maintaining a sense of personal identity in a profession that often consumes every waking hour (and some non-waking ones, too).

In this chapter, we'll explore the importance of hobbies, how they can make you a better surgeon, and practical tips for fitting them into a packed residency schedule. Whether it's painting, playing guitar, or becoming a master of sourdough, your hobbies are a lifeline to balance and sanity.

The Mental Health Benefits of Hobbies

1. **Stress Relief Through Creative Outlets**

    ◆   **Switching Gears:** Engaging in a hobby shifts your brain away from work-related stressors, providing a mental "reset."

- ◆ **Flow State**: Hobbies often induce a flow state, where you're completely absorbed in the activity, leaving no room for stress or intrusive thoughts.

2. **Boosting Mood and Reducing Burnout**

   - ◆ Creative pursuits stimulate the release of endorphins and dopamine, improving mood and countering burnout.

   - ◆ Even simple hobbies like journaling or sketching can serve as emotional outlets.

Interactive Element

✳   Reflect: What hobby or interest always brings you joy, even in small doses? How can you make space for it in your life this week?

....

....

....

Encouraging Residents to Pursue Creative Outlets

1. **Busting the "I Don't Have Time" Myth**

   - ◆ **Micro-Hobbies**: Small, manageable hobbies like reading short stories, doodling, or doing puzzles can fit into even the busiest schedules.

   - ◆ **Time as an Investment**: Spending time on hobbies might feel indulgent, but it pays dividends in mental clarity and focus.

2. **Finding Your Creative Passion**

   - ◆ Explore a variety of activities until you find something that resonates—whether it's photography, gardening, or baking.

   - ◆ Hobbies don't have to be "productive" or "perfect." The joy is in the doing, not the outcome.

Interactive Element

✳   Try this: Dedicate 15 minutes today to a hobby you've always wanted to try. Reflect on how it feels to step away from work for a moment.

Balancing Your Surgical Identity with Your Personal Identity

1. **Avoiding the "Surgical Robot" Trap**

    ◆   Residency can make you feel like you're defined solely by your profession.

    ◆   Developing interests outside medicine reminds you that you're a whole person, not just a title or skill set.

2. **Enriching Your Perspective as a Surgeon**

    ◆   Pursuing hobbies can improve your empathy, creativity, and communication skills, making you a better doctor.

    ◆   A well-rounded identity allows you to connect with patients on a human level, not just a professional one.

Interactive Element

✳   Journal Prompt: How does your personal identity enhance your professional life? List three ways your hobbies or interests make you a better surgeon.

....

....

....

Better Stress Management Through Physical Activities or Meditation.

Pursuing activities like running, yoga, or mindfulness meditation helps in managing stress, improving focus, and maintaining emotional stability during high-pressure situations in the OR.

◆ Benefit: A calm and composed demeanor ensures clear decision-making during emergencies and enhances overall performance under pressure.

Enhanced Empathy and Communication Through Social or Creative Hobbies.

Participating in storytelling, theater, or volunteer activities fosters emotional intelligence and better interpersonal skills. This can improve interactions with patients and their families, making difficult conversations more compassionate and effective.

◆ Benefit: A surgeon who connects with patients empathetically can build trust, which is essential for patient care and recovery.

Practical Tips for Pursuing Hobbies During Residency

1. **Schedule It Like a Surgery**

   ◆ Block time for hobbies on your calendar, just as you would for rounds or OR time.

   ◆ Even 20 minutes of dedicated hobby time can recharge your mental batteries.

2. **Turn Your Commute into a Hobby Opportunity**

   ◆ Audiobooks, podcasts, or language-learning apps can make your daily commute feel like a creative or educational escape.

3. **Involve Your Friends and Family**

   ◆ Sharing a hobby with loved ones can strengthen relationships and make the activity even more enjoyable.

   ▲ Example: Cook a new recipe with a friend or take a quick hike with your partner.

Interactive Element

✳　Challenge: Write down three small steps you can take this week to make time for a hobby. Share your plan with a friend for accountability.

....

....

....

....

Hobbies That Compliment Surgical Skills

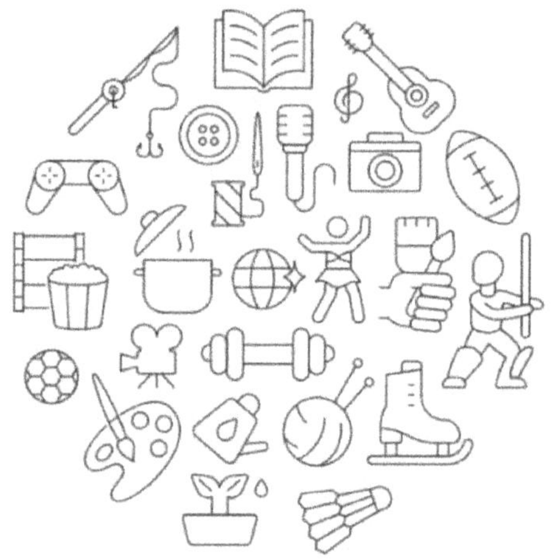

1.　**Fine Motor Skill Hobbies**

◆　Activities like knitting, painting, or playing musical instruments can enhance dexterity and precision.

2.　**Problem-Solving Hobbies**

◆　Puzzles, chess, or even escape rooms sharpen critical thinking and decision-making.

3. **Physical Hobbies**

   ◆ Yoga, martial arts, or dance improve coordination, stamina, and stress management.

Interactive Element

✳ Reflect: What hobby aligns with your strengths as a surgeon? How could you incorporate it into your routine?

....

....

....

✳ "Scrub hands aren't just for surgery—they're also perfect for delicate cookie decorating."

In the whirlwind of residency, it's easy to feel like every minute must be spent advancing your career. But the truth is, the surgeon who cultivates a life outside the OR—filled with hobbies, passions, and joy—is the one who will thrive in the long term. So, go ahead: pick up that paintbrush, lace up those hiking boots, or join that improv class. Your future self (and your patients) will thank you.

Summary: Key Takeaways on Cultivating Hobbies

1. Hobbies are essential for mental well-being and stress relief.

2. Even small hobbies can help shift your mindset and recharge your energy.

3. Creative outlets like painting, writing, or cooking boost mood and foster resilience.

4. Hobbies remind you that you're more than your profession.

5. Sharing hobbies with friends or family enhances your connections and makes the experience more fun.

6. Scheduling hobby time ensures it doesn't get lost in the chaos of residency.

7.　Pursuing hobbies that complement surgical skills can be both relaxing and professionally enriching.

8.　Your hobbies aren't just a luxury—they're a necessity for maintaining balance and sanity.

12

Preparing for Post-Residency Life

Introduction: From Residency to Reality

Congratulations—you've almost crossed the finish line of one of the most grueling journeys in medicine: surgical residency. But as you prepare to enter the next phase, it's important to recognize that post-residency life is not a magical land where stress disappears, and balance effortlessly falls into place. It's a new chapter, one where the choices you make will determine your professional trajectory and personal well-being.

This chapter will guide you in crafting a post-residency life that aligns with both your career ambitions and the lessons you've learned about self-care and mindfulness. With practical advice, humor, and interactive elements, we'll ensure you step out of residency equipped to thrive—not just survive.

Planning a Career That Balances Goals and Well-Being

1. **Defining Your Version of Success**

    ◆   **Avoiding Comparisons:** Your career is yours alone—whether you dream of being a top academic surgeon, a community-based generalist, or something else entirely, own it.

- ◆ **Setting Priorities**: Ask yourself: What matters most? Prestige, financial stability, location, or work-life balance?

2. **Choosing the Right Work Environment**

   - ◆ **Hospital vs. Private Practice**: Understand the pros and cons of different practice settings.

   - ◆ **ulture Matters**: Seek environments that value your well-being as much as your skills.

3. **Negotiating Contracts with Care**

   - ◆ Look beyond salary—consider workload, call schedules, vacation time, and support systems.

   - ◆ Advocate for boundaries: Contracts that respect your time and health are crucial.

Interactive Element

✳ Reflect: Write down your top three career priorities post-residency. How do they align with your vision of a fulfilling life?

Example:

1. Private Practice

2. Mentorship in Medical Education

3. Improving Surgical Skills by Working at Corporate Hospitals

   1. Private Practice

      Pros:

      - ⚔ Autonomy: You have control over your schedule, patient care, and decision-making.

      - ⚔ Higher Earning Potential: Depending on the location and patient base, private practice can offer higher financial rewards.

      - ⚔ Personalized Care: Allows for a more patient-centered approach with better continuity of care.

- ⮞ Flexibility: Ability to set your work hours and design a work-life balance that suits your lifestyle.

- ⮞ Reputation Building: Directly managing your practice helps you build a name in the community.

Cons:

- ⮞ Financial Risk: High upfront investment for infrastructure, equipment, and staff.

- ⮞ Administrative Burden: Requires managing business operations, including billing, marketing, and hiring staff.

- ⮞ Competition: Building a patient base in a competitive area can be challenging.

- ⮞ Isolation: Lack of interaction with peers compared to working in group or academic settings.

- ⮞ Workload: Running a practice can be demanding and time-consuming, especially in the initial years.

2. Mentorship in Medical Education

Pros:

- ⮞ Legacy Building: Opportunity to shape the next generation of surgeons and leave a lasting impact.

- ⮞ Personal Growth: Teaching sharpens your own surgical and communication skills.

- ⮞ Networking: Builds relationships with students, residents, and academic peers.

- ⮞ Job Satisfaction: Mentorship can be deeply fulfilling as you help others grow in their careers.

- ⮞ Career Advancement: Teaching roles often lead to leadership opportunities in academic settings.

Cons:

- ⮞ Time-Consuming: Balancing mentorship with clinical duties can be challenging.

- Institutional Limitations: Working in academic settings may involve bureaucracy and limitations on innovative approaches.

- Lower Pay: Salaries in teaching hospitals or academic institutions are often lower than in private practice or corporate hospitals.

- Burnout Risk: Mentorship responsibilities can add to the overall workload and stress.

3. Improving Surgical Skills by Working at Corporate Hospitals

Pros:

- Access to Advanced Technology: Exposure to state-of-the-art surgical tools, robotic systems, and cutting-edge techniques.

- Diverse and Complex Cases: Opportunity to handle a variety of challenging surgical cases that enhance expertise.

- Multidisciplinary Collaboration: Working with highly skilled teams provides valuable learning and networking opportunities.

- Financial Benefits: Competitive salaries, bonuses, and benefits are common in corporate hospitals.

- Professional Development: Hospitals often provide funding for certifications, workshops, and conferences.

Cons:

- Less Autonomy: Corporate hospitals may impose strict protocols, guidelines, and schedules.

- High Expectations: Pressure to meet performance metrics, such as patient volume and surgical outcomes.

- Workload: High patient turnover and demanding schedules can lead to burnout.

⚔ Limited Patient Relationships: Less continuity of care compared to private practice, as patients may be referred to multiple specialists.

⚔ Corporate Influence: Decisions may be driven by hospital policies or profitability rather than patient-centric care.

⚔ "Remember, the dream job isn't worth it if you're too busy working to spend your paycheck."

Transitioning with Healthy Coping Mechanisms

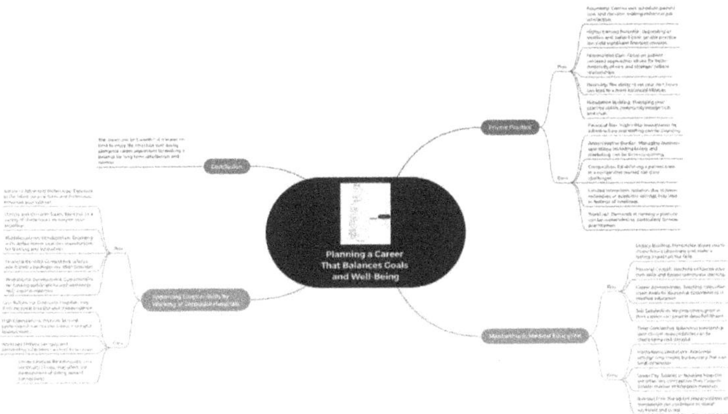

1. **Managing the Emotional Shift**

   ◆ **Post-Residency Blues**: Many feel a strange sense of loss or disorientation after the structured chaos of residency. It's normal.

   ◆ **Celebrate Milestones**: Take time to acknowledge what you've achieved—plan a vacation, throw a party, or simply reflect on how far you've come.

2. **Building a Sustainable Routine**

   ◆ **Redefining Productivity**: Without the constant demands of residency, you'll need to find a rhythm that feels productive but not overwhelming.

◆ **Carve Out Time for Wellness**: Ensure your schedule includes regular exercise, mindfulness practices, and hobbies.

3. **Financial Wellness**

◆ **Managing Debt**: Work with a financial planner to prioritize loan repayment while building savings.

◆ **Invest in Your Future**: Start planning for long-term financial goals, such as retirement or buying a home.

Interactive Element

✳ Activity: Write down one thing you'll do differently post-residency to ensure your well-being remains a priority.

Fostering Relationships and Support Systems

1. **Strengthening Personal Relationships**

◆ **Reconnect**: Residency often strains relationships. Use this time to reconnect with family and friends.

◆ **Quality Time**: Make an effort to be fully present during personal moments—put away your phone and truly engage.

2. **Professional Support Networks**

◆ **Mentorship**: Continue to seek guidance from trusted mentors as you navigate new challenges.

◆ **Peer Connections**: Build a community of colleagues who understand the unique pressures of surgery.

3. **Setting Boundaries to Protect Your Time**

◆ Learn to say NO: Protecting your personal time isn't selfish; it's essential.

◆ Practice delegation: You don't have to do it all. Lean on your team when appropriate.

Interactive Element

✳ Prompt: Identify one relationship (personal or professional) you'd like to nurture post-residency. Write down three actions you'll take to strengthen it.

1. ....

2. ....

3. ....

Mindfulness and Self-Reflection Post-Residency

1. **Reflect on Lessons Learned**

   ◆ What worked for you during residency? What didn't? Use these insights to shape your approach moving forward.

   ◆ Journaling can help clarify your goals and provide a sense of direction.

2. **Staying Present in the Moment**

   ◆ Avoid falling into the trap of "I'll be happy when..." thinking.

   ◆ Mindfulness exercises, such as breathing techniques, can help you appreciate the journey as much as the destination.

3. **Embracing Change with Confidence**

   ◆ Post-residency life is a big adjustment, but it's also an opportunity for growth.

   ◆ Approach challenges with curiosity rather than fear—you've already survived the toughest part!

Interactive Element

✳ Try this: Spend five minutes today visualizing your ideal post-residency life. Focus on how it feels to achieve balance and fulfillment.

✱   "If you can survive a 24-hour call, you can survive figuring out post-residency paperwork."

Residency has been an incredible training ground, not just for surgery but for resilience, determination, and adaptability. As you step into this new phase, remember that the same skills that carried you through sleepless nights and difficult cases will guide you now. With a clear vision, a strong support system, and a commitment to your well-being, you can craft a post-residency life that's as fulfilling as it is impactful.

Summary: Key Takeaways for Preparing for Post-Residency Life

1.   Define success on your terms—don't let others dictate your goals.

2.   Choose a work environment that aligns with your values and priorities.

3.   Post-residency life can feel disorienting; give yourself time to adjust.

4.   Celebrate your achievements—it's okay to enjoy the moment.

5.   Build a routine that includes wellness practices like mindfulness and exercise.

6.   Strengthen personal relationships and professional networks for support.

7.   Financial planning is essential—start early to secure your future.

8.   Embrace change with confidence and stay present in your journey.

13

Conclusion – Steady Hands, Steady Mind

Introduction: The Journey Doesn't End Here

Congratulations, dear reader. If you've made it this far, you've traversed a roadmap for navigating the high-stress, high-stakes world of surgical residency and beyond. But let's be clear: the lessons in this book aren't meant to be tucked away like an old textbook. They're your tools for a lifetime.

In surgery, as in life, steadiness is key—not just in the precision of your hands but in the clarity of your mind. This chapter will recap key takeaways from the book, provide final encouragement, and offer a reminder that mindfulness and well-being are lifelong pursuits.

Recap of Key Takeaways

1. **Understanding the Realities of Residency**

   ◆ Residency is tough, but acknowledging the challenges is the first step toward resilience.

   ◆ "Remember, every sleepless night is just a future humblebrag: 'Back in my residency days…'"

2. **Embracing Mindfulness**

   ◆ Mindfulness isn't just a trend—it's a scientifically proven method to improve focus, patience, and stress management.

   ◆ Practical Insight: If you can find a moment of mindfulness in the chaos of the OR, you can find it anywhere.

3. **Practical Techniques for Mindfulness and Stress Management**

   ◆ Whether it's deep breathing between cases or a quiet moment during rounds, small practices add up.

   ◆ "When in doubt, breathe. If nothing else, it buys you time to come up with a better response."

4. **Physical and Mental Health Are Non-Negotiable**

   ◆ A well-maintained body supports a sharp mind. Regular exercise, sleep hygiene, and balanced nutrition aren't luxuries—they're necessities.

5. **Relationships Matter**

   ◆ Support systems are lifelines. Lean on your mentors, peers, and loved ones when the going gets tough.

6. **Work-Life Balance Is a Skill**

   ◆ Learning to say NO and setting boundaries is an act of self-preservation, not selfishness.

The Ongoing Journey of Mindfulness

1. **Mindfulness as a Career-Long Practice**

   ◆ Residency was just the beginning. The demands of a surgical career mean you'll need to continually adapt your mindfulness and self-care strategies.

   ◆ Schedule mindfulness like you'd schedule a meeting. Consistency is key.

2. **Avoiding Burnout Through Intentionality**

    ◆ Burnout isn't a single event—it's a process. Recognizing the early signs can save your career and your health.

    ◆ Use reflective journaling to assess your emotional and physical state regularly.

3. **Redefining Success Over Time**

    ◆ Your definition of success will evolve. Be open to reassessing and realigning your goals.

    ◆ "Success is flexible. Today it's a perfectly sutured anastomosis; tomorrow it's 8 hours of sleep."

Interactive Element

* Exercise: Write down one mindfulness habit you want to commit to for the next month. What small step can you take today to make it happen?

....

Prioritizing Mental and Physical Well-Being

1. **The Surgeon's Toolbox for Health**

    ◆ **Physical Health**: Never underestimate the power of a strong body to support a sharp mind.

    ◆ **Mental Health**: Therapy, mindfulness, and peer support are invaluable tools—not signs of weakness.

2. **Self-Care Beyond the OR**

    ◆ Pursue hobbies, spend time with loved ones, and allow yourself moments of joy outside medicine.

    ◆ "Remember, you're not just a surgeon; you're also a human who occasionally needs to binge-watch Netflix."

3. **Sharing the Load**

    ◆   You're not alone in this journey. Rely on your colleagues, mentors, and loved ones.

    ◆   Organize regular debriefs with peers to share challenges and solutions.

Encouragement for the Journey Ahead

1. **Trust in Your Growth**

    ◆   Look at how far you've come. You've survived grueling nights, tough cases, and impossible schedules. You're equipped to face what lies ahead.

    ◆   "If you can handle a 3 a.m. emergency laparotomy, you can handle a bit of work-life balance."

2. **Keep Evolving**

    ◆   The surgeon you are today is not the surgeon you'll be tomorrow. Embrace change with an open mind and a steady heart.

3. **Remember Why You Started**

    ◆   Amid the chaos, hold onto the core of why you chose this path—to help, to heal, to make a difference.

Interactive Element

*   Reflect: Write a letter to your future self, reminding yourself of the lessons and commitments you want to carry forward.

Summary: Key Takeaways

1. **Residency Lessons**: Acknowledge the challenges of residency but use them to build resilience.

2. **Mindfulness**: Incorporate mindfulness into your daily life for focus and stress reduction.

3. **Physical Health**: Exercise, eat well, and sleep regularly to maintain stamina and clarity.

4. **Mental Health**: Seek therapy, support systems, and self-care routines when needed.

5. **Boundaries**: Protect your personal time to sustain long-term productivity and happiness.

6. **Relationships**: Build strong support networks with mentors, peers, and loved ones.

7. **Work-Life Balance**: Balance isn't a myth; it's a skill you can cultivate over time.

8. **Long-Term Success**: Reassess and redefine success as your career evolves.

9. **Continuous Growth**: Embrace change and remain open to learning.

10. **Gratitude**: Always remember why you chose this journey and stay grounded in your purpose.

Final Thought: A Life Well Lived

In the end, surgery is as much about the mind as it is about the hands. The best surgeons are those who master not just the art of healing others but the skill of caring for themselves. You've been given the tools to forge a career of impact, balance, and fulfillment. Use them wisely, and remember: a steady mind makes for steady hands.

As you step into the next phase of your career, take this book as your companion, a reminder that no matter how high the stakes, you are capable of achieving both excellence and peace.